Colorectal Cancer Screening

It's easy to get lost in the cancer world

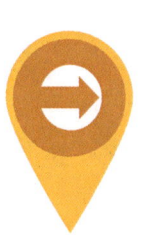

Let
NCCN Guidelines for Patients®
be your guide

✓ Step-by-step guides to the cancer care options likely to have the best results

✓ Based on treatment guidelines used by health care providers worldwide

✓ Designed to help you discuss cancer treatment with your doctors

Colorectal Cancer Screening

National Comprehensive Cancer Network®

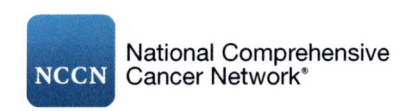

NCCN Guidelines for Patients® are developed by the National Comprehensive Cancer Network® (NCCN®)

NCCN

- ✓ An alliance of leading cancer centers across the United States devoted to patient care, research, and education

Cancer centers that are part of NCCN:
NCCN.org/cancercenters

NCCN Clinical Practice Guidelines in Oncology (NCCN Guidelines®)

- ✓ Developed by doctors from NCCN cancer centers using the latest research and years of experience
- ✓ For providers of cancer care all over the world
- ✓ Expert recommendations for cancer screening, diagnosis, and treatment

Free online at
NCCN.org/guidelines

NCCN Guidelines for Patients

- ✓ Present information from the NCCN Guidelines in an easy-to-learn format
- ✓ For people with cancer and those who support them
- ✓ Explain the cancer care options likely to have the best results

Free online at
NCCN.org/patientguidelines

These NCCN Guidelines for Patients are based on the NCCN Guidelines® for Colorectal Cancer Screening, Version 2.2021 – April 13, 2021.

© 2021 National Comprehensive Cancer Network, Inc. All rights reserved. NCCN Guidelines for Patients and illustrations herein may not be reproduced in any form for any purpose without the express written permission of NCCN. No one, including doctors or patients, may use the NCCN Guidelines for Patients for any commercial purpose and may not claim, represent, or imply that the NCCN Guidelines for Patients that have been modified in any manner are derived from, based on, related to, or arise out of the NCCN Guidelines for Patients. The NCCN Guidelines are a work in progress that may be redefined as often as new significant data become available. NCCN makes no warranties of any kind whatsoever regarding its content, use, or application and disclaims any responsibility for its application or use in any way.

NCCN Foundation seeks to support the millions of patients and their families affected by a cancer diagnosis by funding and distributing NCCN Guidelines for Patients. NCCN Foundation is also committed to advancing cancer treatment by funding the nation's promising doctors at the center of innovation in cancer research. For more details and the full library of patient and caregiver resources, visit NCCN.org/patients.

National Comprehensive Cancer Network (NCCN) / NCCN Foundation
3025 Chemical Road, Suite 100
Plymouth Meeting, PA 19462
215.690.0300

NCCN Guidelines for Patients®
Colorectal Cancer Screening, 2021

Colorectal Cancer Screening

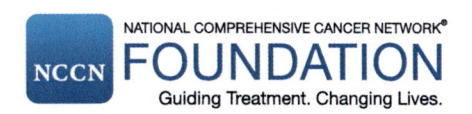

NCCN Guidelines for Patients are supported by funding from the NCCN Foundation®

To make a gift or learn more, please visit NCCNFoundation.org/donate or e-mail PatientGuidelines@NCCN.org.

Also supported by Fight Colorectal Cancer

We fight to cure colorectal cancer and serve as relentless champions of hope for all affected by this disease through informed patient support, impactful policy change, and breakthrough research endeavors. As an organization dedicated to helping the community find trusted resources to make informed decisions about their health, we are proud to support this comprehensive resource.
Fightcolorectalcancer.org

With generous support from:

Kristina Gregory
Lois & Donald Howland
John Kisiel
Wui-Jin Koh
Elizabeth & Brian Rizor
Marianne & Gary Weyhmuller

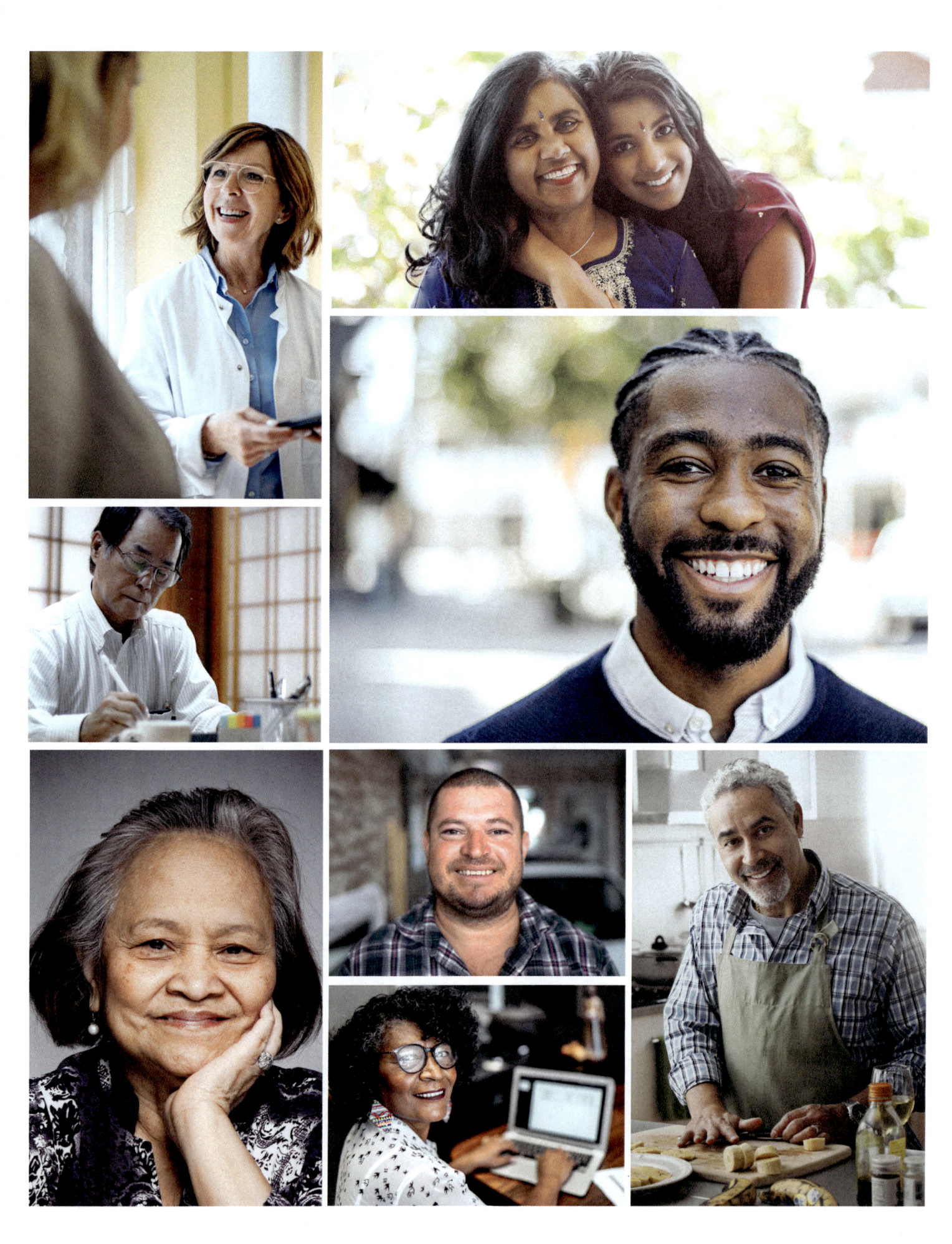

NCCN Guidelines for Patients®
Colorectal Cancer Screening, 2021

Colorectal Cancer Screening

Contents

6 Cancer screening saves lives

14 Average risk of colorectal cancer

20 Family health history

26 Colorectal polyps and cancer

33 Inflammatory bowel disease

39 Resources

40 Words to know

43 NCCN Contributors

44 NCCN Cancer Centers

46 Index

1
Cancer screening saves lives

7 What is colorectal cancer?
9 Why get screened?
10 Who should get screened?
12 What saves lives besides screening?
13 Key points

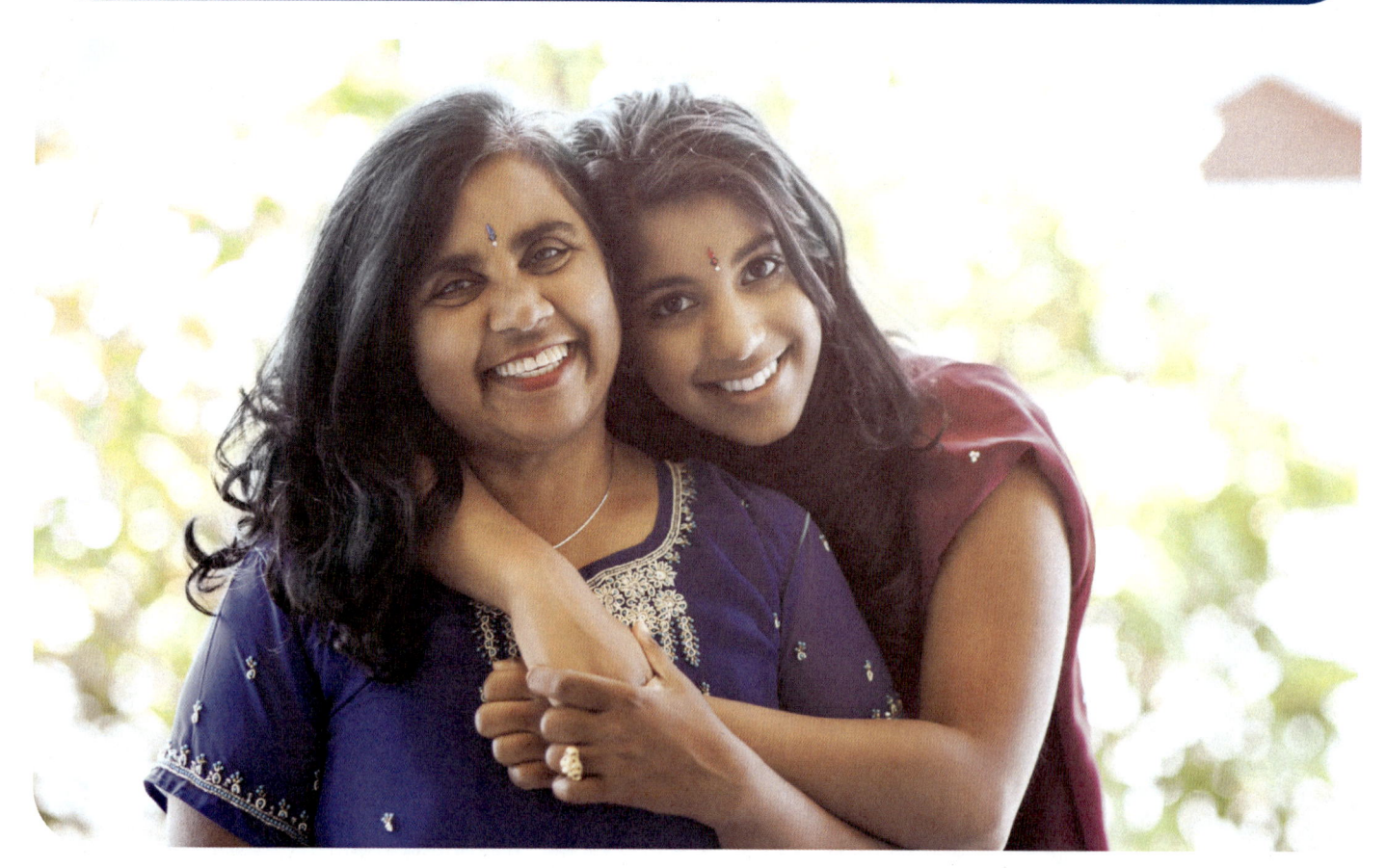

1 Cancer screening saves lives | What is colorectal cancer?

Colorectal cancer is the third most common cancer in the world. Screening can prevent colorectal cancer and find it early when a cure is more likely.

What is colorectal cancer?

The human body is made of over 30 trillion cells. Cancer is a disease of abnormal cells that grow out of control. Colorectal cancer refers to cancer of the colon or rectum.

The colon and rectum are organs in the digestive system

The digestive system breaks down food for the body to use. In the stomach, food is broken down into small pieces. In the small intestine, almost all the nutrients from food are absorbed into the bloodstream.

The digestive system also removes undigested food from the body. In the large intestine, water and salts are removed from undigested food as it passes through the colon. Solid food waste is called feces or stool. The rectum holds stool until it exits the body through an opening called the anus.

Some polyps progress into colorectal cancer

The colorectal wall is made of layers of tissue. The innermost layer that comes in contact with stool is called the mucosa. Areas of abnormal cell growth, called polyps, commonly occur in the mucosa.

Colon and rectum

The colon and rectum are part of the large intestine. The colon is the longest part—about 5 feet (1½ meters) long. It has four sections: ascending, transverse, descending, and sigmoid colon. The rectum is near the end of the large intestine. It is about 5 inches (12 centimeters) long.

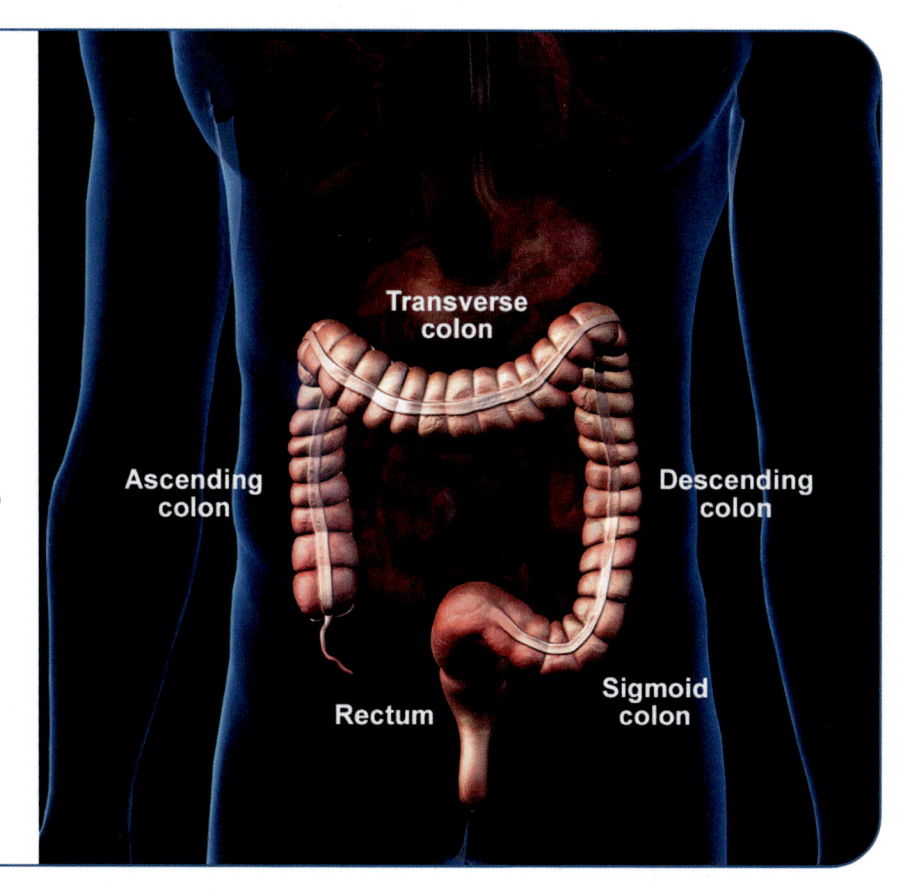

| 1 Cancer screening saves lives | What is colorectal cancer? |

While most polyps do not become cancer, almost all colorectal cancers start as polyps. There are different types of polyps, and some are more likely to become cancer than others. It takes many years for a polyp to transform into a cancer.

Cancer cells have uncontrolled growth

When cells become cancerous, they don't behave like normal cells. They break the rules of normal cell growth.

> Unlike normal cells, cancer cells don't die when they should. They also make many new cancer cells that replace normal cells over time.

> Cancer cells don't stay in place. They can grow through the colorectal wall and into nearby organs and tissues.

> Cancer cells can spread to other parts of the body. Blood and lymph vessels are inside the colorectal wall. Once the cancer cells have reached these vessels, they can spread.

A staging system is a standard way of grouping cancers by their growth and spread. The stages of colorectal cancer range from stage 0 to stage 4. The more serious the cancer growth and spread, the higher the stage.

As cancer grows, it can cause symptoms. When there are symptoms, cancer is usually advanced and harder to cure. If treatment doesn't work, cancer cells will keep growing and cause organs to stop working.

Colon and rectal polyps

Polyps are lesions that grow in the colorectal wall. They have many shapes. Raised polyps that look like a mushroom are called pedunculated polyps (left). Sessile polyps have a round top and wide base (right).

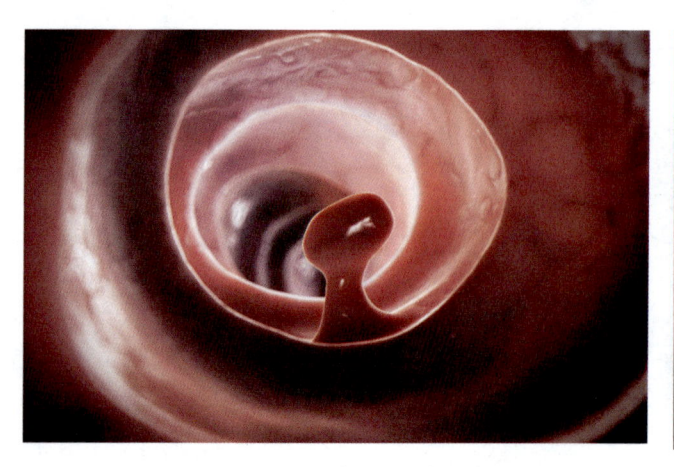

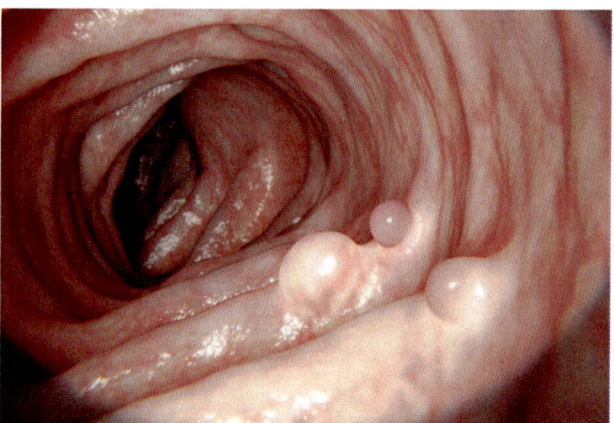

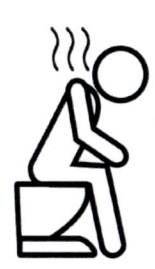

| 1 | Cancer screening saves lives | Why get screened? |

Why get screened?

Colorectal cancer screening looks for polyps and cancer before symptoms start. It saves lives in two ways:

> **Screening prevents colorectal cancer.** Cancer is prevented when polyps are removed before they become cancer.

> **Screening finds cancer early before symptoms start.** When cancer is found early, it is easier to treat or cure.

Screening is started when a person is at risk for colorectal cancer. There are several screening methods:

> **Endoscopy** involves a hand-held device that allows doctors, such as gastroenterologists, to look inside the colon and rectum for abnormal growths.

> **Imaging** makes pictures of the inside of the colon and rectum. A radiologist will review the pictures for abnormal growths.

> **Lab tests** find cancer markers, such as blood, in stool.

The only screening method that can remove polyps is endoscopy. Endoscopic procedures for colorectal cancer screening are colonoscopy and flexible sigmoidoscopy.

The removed polyps will be sent to an expert called a pathologist. This doctor will look for cancer cells in the polyp using a microscope. If cancer cells are found, a cancer diagnosis is made.

Screening vs. diagnosis

Cancer screening is done if you have no signs or symptoms of colorectal cancer. Once you have signs or symptoms, the aim of testing is to find the problem and make a diagnosis. Ask your health care provider about getting colorectal cancer screening right away if you have these signs or symptoms:

Iron-deficiency anemia

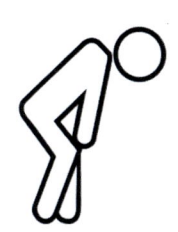

Bloody stools

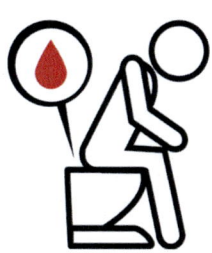

Change in bowel habits

NCCN Guidelines for Patients®
Colorectal Cancer Screening, 2021

1 Cancer screening saves lives | Who should get screened?

Who should get screened?

Risk is the chance that an event will occur. Risk is part of life. There are risks when we eat, travel, and invest money. Life also includes a risk of health problems, including cancer.

Some people are more likely to get colorectal cancer than others

Things that increase risk are called risk factors. For example, a risk factor of getting a cold is close contact with an infected person.

There are many risk factors of colorectal cancer. Some can be changed, such as:

- Eating highly processed food
- Smoking
- Not exercising

Other risk factors can't be changed, such as:

- Your age
- Your health history

If you have risk factors, it doesn't mean you are certain to get colorectal cancer. Similarly, you can get colorectal cancer even if you have no known risk factors.

Some risk factors affect the timing of cancer screening

Not all risk factors have the same effect. **See Guide 1** for risk levels that are used to tailor colorectal cancer screening for each person.

Learn what your risk of colorectal cancer is before age 40, so you don't start screening late. Learn your risk sooner if your family has had colorectal cancer.

Guide 1. Risk levels of colorectal cancer

Average risk	You are at least 45 years of age and have no other major risk factors
Increased risk	Your family by birth has a history of colorectal cancer or advanced pre-cancer polyps
	You have had colorectal cancer or polyps that increase cancer risk
	You have either one of these inflammatory bowel diseases: • Ulcerative colitis • Crohn's colitis
High risk	You have one of these hereditary cancer syndromes: • Lynch syndrome • Polyposis syndromes, such as classical and attenuated familial adenomatous polyposis

1 Cancer screening saves lives | Who should get screened?

The time to start colorectal cancer screening and be rescreened is discussed in the next chapters.

- Chapter 2 covers screening for people with average risk.
- Chapter 3 discusses screening when there is family history of colorectal cancer or pre-cancer polyps. It also briefly discusses hereditary cancer syndromes.
- Chapter 4 explains rescreening if you've had pre-cancer polyps or colorectal cancer.
- Chapter 5 explains the screening process if you have inflammatory bowel disease.

"

Colorectal cancer screening is SO important! Colorectal cancer is one of the few cancers that is not only highly treatable when detected early, but can actually be prevented with regular screening! While the preparation for a colonoscopy, or the process of collecting a sample for an at-home screening test may seem off-putting, I can promise you, as a stage III colon cancer survivor, they are much preferable to colorectal cancer treatments like radiation and chemotherapy!

– Ben

1 Cancer screening saves lives | What saves lives besides screening?

What saves lives besides screening?

Screening is important for preventing colorectal cancer. There are 7 other actions you can take to prevent colorectal cancer:

1. Take aspirin

Taking aspirin every day for at least 5 to 10 years protects against developing colorectal cancer. Ask your health care provider if aspirin is right for you. Internal bleeding is a risk of taking aspirin.

2. Eat healthful foods

- Eat lots of plant-based foods.
- Eat limited amounts of red meat and avoid processed meat.
- Limit eating of processed and ultra-processed foods.
- Don't rely on dietary supplements alone for nutrients. Get nutrients from natural food.

3. Drink little to no alcohol

High and moderate drinking of alcohol may increase the risk of colorectal cancer. The amount of alcohol that is safe depends on a person's biology. The risk of colon cancer does not increase with 1 drink a day for women and 2 drinks a day for men.

4. Move more and rest less often

Physical activity on a regular basis has been linked with a lower risk of colorectal cancer.

5. Get enough vitamin D

Low levels of vitamin D may increase the risk of colorectal cancer. Prevent low levels by eating foods with vitamin D. Vitamin D is in salmon, tuna, mackerel, and egg yolks. You can also eat vitamin D-fortified foods and take supplements.

Your skin can make vitamin D when exposed to the sun. Sunscreen is advised when outside for an extended period of time. Wearing sunscreen may limit the amount of vitamin D made by the skin.

6. Maintain a healthy weight

Obesity is another risk factor of colorectal cancer. A body mass index (BMI) is a measure of body fat. A BMI of 18.5 to 24.9 is considered normal weight. Tracking your weight, diet, calories, and activity levels may help you meet your goals.

7. Quit smoking

If you smoke, quit! Ask your health care providers for help to quit. There is counseling for quitting smoking. Medication can help to stop cravings and withdrawal symptoms.

1 Cancer screening saves lives | Key points

Key points

- Colorectal cancer refers to cancer of the colon or rectum. These two organs are part of the digestive system. They help remove stool from the body.

- Polyps are an overgrowth of the inner lining of the colon or rectum. While most polyps do not become cancer, almost all colorectal cancers start as polyps.

- Colorectal cancer screening saves lives. It prevents cancer by finding and removing polyps before they become cancer. It also finds cancer early when a cure is more likely.

- Risk is the chance that an event will occur. A risk of cancer is part of life for everyone.

- Things that increase risk are called risk factors. There are many risk factors of colorectal cancer.

- Some risk factors increase the risk of colorectal cancer more than others. Risk factors that affect the timing of colorectal cancer screening include age and health. Risk of colorectal cancer is grouped by average, increased, and high risk.

- Taking aspirin and living a healthy lifestyle can help prevent colorectal cancer in addition to cancer screening.

Cancer won't wait and neither should you

During the COVID-19 pandemic, the number of people getting recommended cancer screenings has dropped. Missed screenings may lead to late diagnoses and missed chances for a cure.

Don't wait and neglect routine health care. Take care of yourself by doing routine cancer screenings. Talk to your doctor about when and how often to be screened.

More on NCCN's message that "Cancer Won't Wait and Neither Should You" can be found at NCCN.org/resume-screening.

2 Average risk of colorectal cancer

15 Screening starts at age 45
16 There are screening options
18 The next screen may be in 10 years
19 Key points

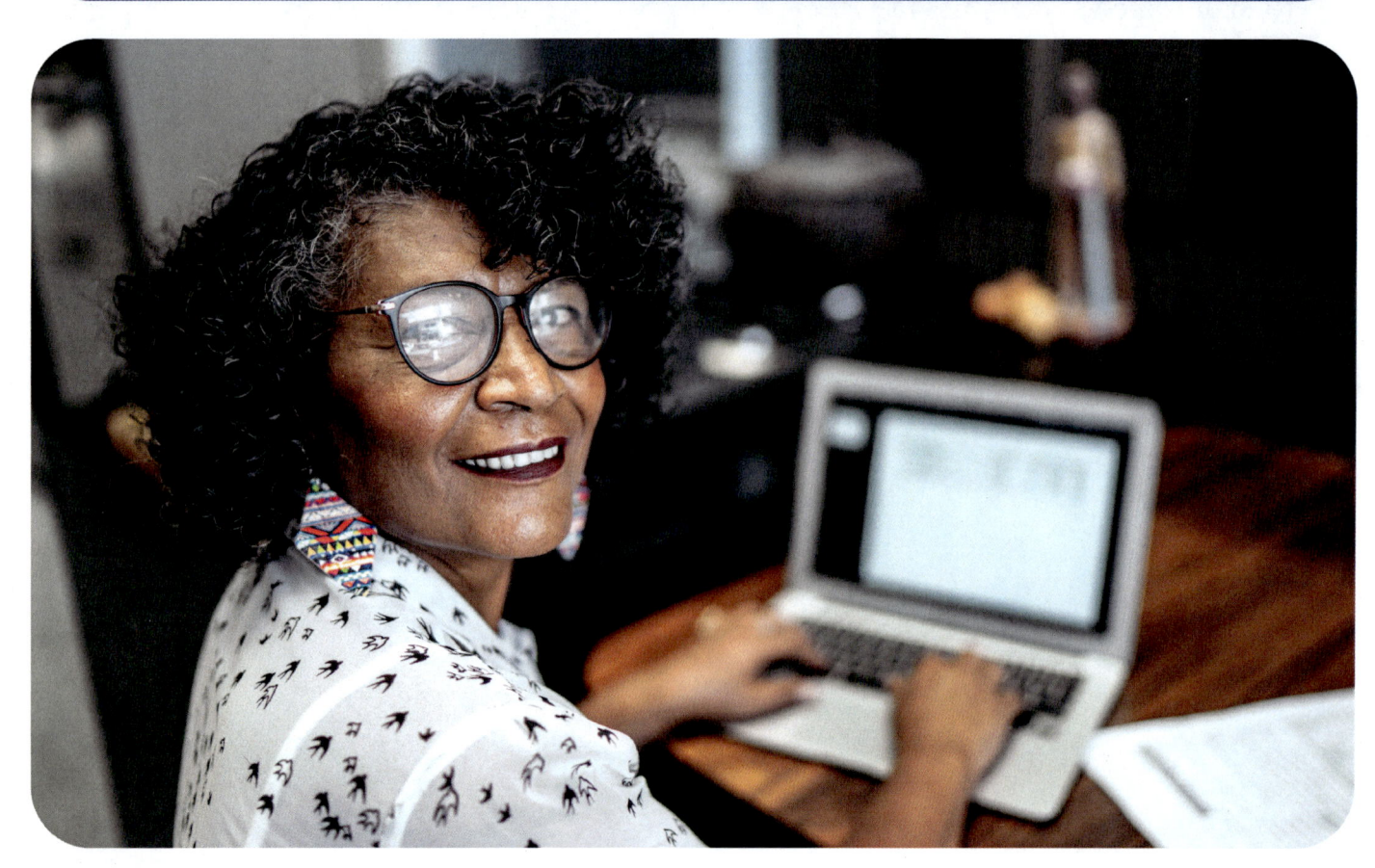

2 Average risk of colorectal cancer | Screening starts at age 45

Most people at risk of colorectal cancer have an average risk. Average risk is based on age and the absence of other major risk factors.

Screening starts at age 45

For years, people with average risk began colorectal cancer screening at 50 years of age. But, colorectal cancer is on the rise in people under 50 years of age. Now, people at average risk start screening at 45 years of age.

The risk of colorectal cancer differs by ethnicity and race. In the United States, the highest rates of colorectal cancer occur among Black individuals. Black individuals should begin screening for colorectal cancer by age 45 or earlier if colorectal cancer runs in the family.

Some people under 45 years of age get colorectal cancer. Some have an increased or high risk of colorectal cancer, but others have no major risk factors. Talk with your health care provider about whether you should start cancer screening before age 45.

People in good health should undergo colorectal cancer screening up to age 75. If you are between 76 and 85 years of age, cancer screening is a personal decision to be made after talking with your health care provider. Ask about the pros and cons of screening in light of your health. Colorectal cancer screening is not needed if you are over 85 years of age.

Ages 45 to 75
Get screened (unless you have a major life-threatening illness).

Ages 76 to 85
Screening is a personal decision. Learn what the pros and cons are for you.

Ages 86 and above
Screening is not needed.

NCCN Guidelines for Patients®
Colorectal Cancer Screening, 2021

There are screening options

People with an average risk of colorectal cancer have several screening options. The best screen is the one you get done. Any screen is better than no screen. Ask your doctor about the pros and cons of each screening option.

Visual screening

Visual screening uses medical devices that allow doctors to see inside your body. It includes colonoscopy, flexible sigmoidoscopy, and computed tomography (CT) colonography. Colonoscopy is needed if there are abnormal findings with flexible sigmoidoscopy or CT colonography.

Visual screening requires that your bowel be cleared of stool. Bowel prep consists of a liquid diet and strong laxatives. Follow your doctor's prep instructions before screening. If your bowel isn't clear enough, you may have to reschedule, repeat the test, or do a different test.

A biopsy is a procedure that removes tissue samples for further testing. A polypectomy is a type of biopsy that removes entire polyps (overgrowths of the inner bowel wall). A biopsy can only be performed during colonoscopy and flexible sigmoidoscopy. A cutting tool is inserted through the endoscope to remove tissue. Most polyps can be removed with an endoscope. Rarely, surgery is needed.

Stool-based screening

Stool-based screening is easier to have than visual tests. At home, you will collect a sample of your stool in a container. You will then send

Colonoscopy

Colonoscopy is a procedure that allows doctors to see inside the bowel. You will be sedated during the procedure. Your doctor will use a hand-held device called an endoscope. Endoscopes designed for colonoscopy are referred to as colonoscopes. Only the thin, tube-shaped part of the device is guided through the anus, up the rectum, and into the colon. The device has a light, a camera, and a cutting tool.

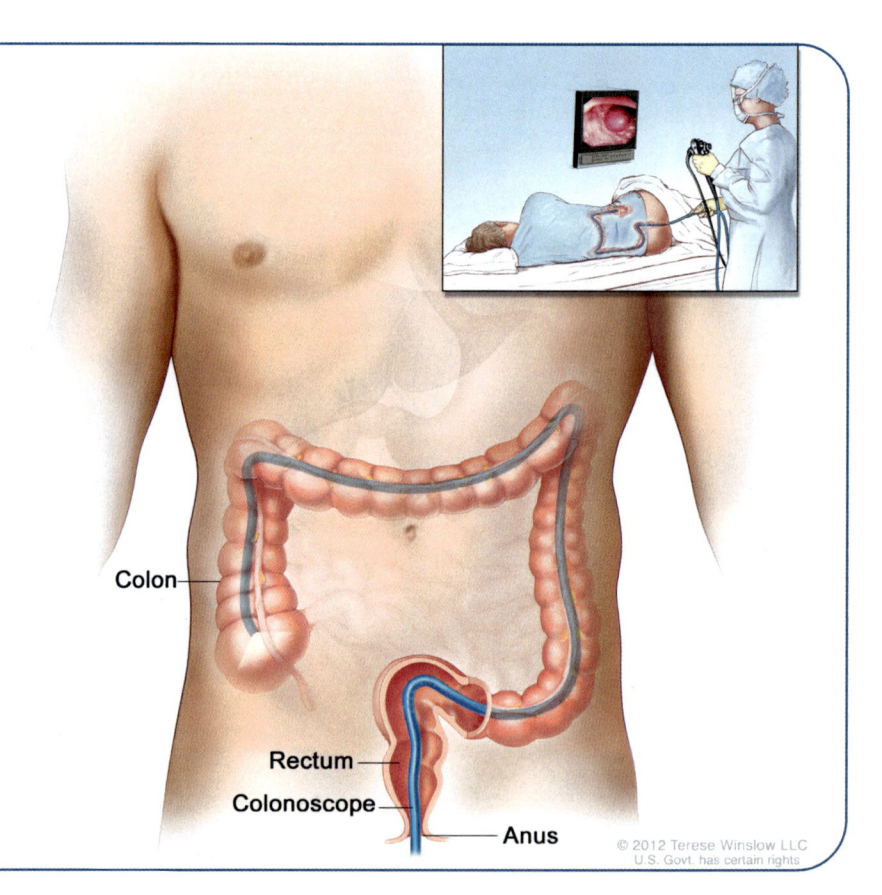

2 Average risk of colorectal cancer | There are screening options

Screening options for average risk

Visual screening	Pros 👍	Cons 👎
Colonoscopy An exam of the colon and rectum with a thin device that is gently inserted through the anus	• One-step screening—no additional test is needed • Very long intervals between screens if findings are normal	• Bowel prep is needed • Completed away from home • Sedation is used • Small risk of bleeding, infection, and injury
Flexible sigmoidoscopy An exam of the last part of the colon with a thin device that is gently inserted through the anus	• Long intervals between screens if findings are normal • Sedation is not needed	• Bowel prep is needed • Completed away from home • Doesn't assess the whole colon • A colonoscopy is needed if polyps are found
CT colonography X-rays of the colon	• Long intervals between screens if findings are normal • Sedation is not needed	• Bowel prep is needed • Completed away from home • May miss flat polyps • Rescreen or a colonoscopy is needed if polyps are found

Stool-based screening		
Multitargeted stool DNA-based test (mt-sDNA) A lab test that looks for genetic markers of cancer in stool **High-sensitivity guaiac-based test and fecal immunochemical test (FIT)** Lab tests that look for tiny amounts of blood in stool	• Stool is collected by you at home • No prep is needed • No physical risks	• A colonoscopy is needed if results are abnormal • Not as accurate as visual tests • Frequent screenings even if results are normal

NCCN Guidelines for Patients®
Colorectal Cancer Screening, 2021

| 2 | Average risk of colorectal cancer | The next screen may be in 10 years |

the sample to a lab for testing. Stool tests include the fecal immunochemical test (FIT), high-sensitivity fecal occult blood test, and multitargeted stool DNA (mt-sDNA) test.

Although easier, stool tests are not as good as visual tests at finding the polyps that become cancer. In addition, screening is a two-step process if stool test results are abnormal. The second step is to receive a colonoscopy within 6 to 10 months of the stool test. No further testing is needed if the colonoscopy findings after FIT or mt-sDNA are normal.

The next screen may be in 10 years

When screening results are normal, the next screening can be done with any screening method. The time interval between screenings varies based on the prior screening method. **See Guide 2** for average-risk screening intervals.

Rescreening with colonoscopy has the longest interval of 10 years. Rescreening with flexible sigmoidoscopy may be done in 10 years if you do the FIT stool test every year.

The interval after visual screening may be adjusted based on the quality of the prior screen. A 1-year interval may be needed if your bowel wasn't cleared enough or the procedure wasn't completed.

If you get pre-cancer polyps or colorectal cancer, read Chapter 4 to learn about the next steps.

Guide 2. Rescreening based on average risk

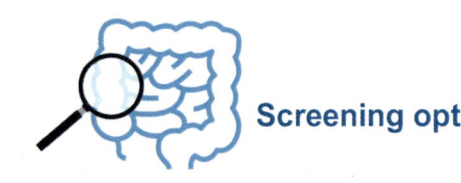

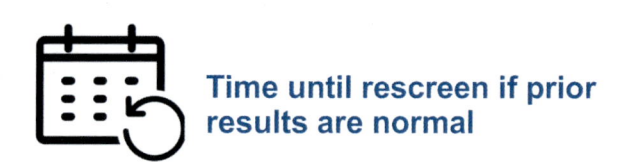

Screening options	Time until rescreen if prior results are normal
Colonoscopy	Rescreen in 10 years
Flexible sigmoidoscopy	Rescreen in 5 to 10 years
CT colonography	Rescreen in 5 years
Multitargeted stool DNA-based test	Rescreen in 3 years
High-sensitivity guaiac-based test	Rescreen in 1 year
Fecal immunochemical test	Rescreen in 1 year

2 Average risk of colorectal cancer | Key points

Key points

- People with an average risk of colorectal cancer start screening at 45 years of age. You must not have any other major risk factors.

- You can choose which type of screening to receive.

- The best screening test is the one you get. Discuss the pros and cons of each screening method with your health care provider so you can make an informed choice.

- The time until the next screening varies based on the prior screening method. Screening is not needed for another 10 years if you have normal results with a colonoscopy. Rescreening after stool tests ranges from 1 to 3 years.

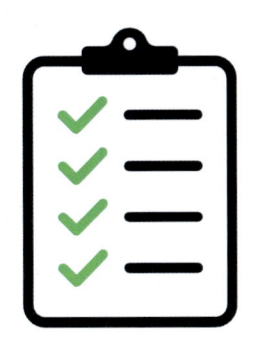

We want your feedback!

Our goal is to provide helpful and easy-to-understand information on cancer.

Take our survey to let us know what we got right and what we could do better:

NCCN.org/patients/feedback

"

Colorectal cancer has always been thought of as an "old person's disease." Now, studies have shown that a person born on or after 1990 is 2 to 4 times more likely to develop colorectal cancer compared to a person born in 1950. Because of this, it is very important to get screened at 45 years old.

– Lara, Rectal cancer survivor

3
Family health history

21 History with high risk
23 History with increased risk
24 Key points

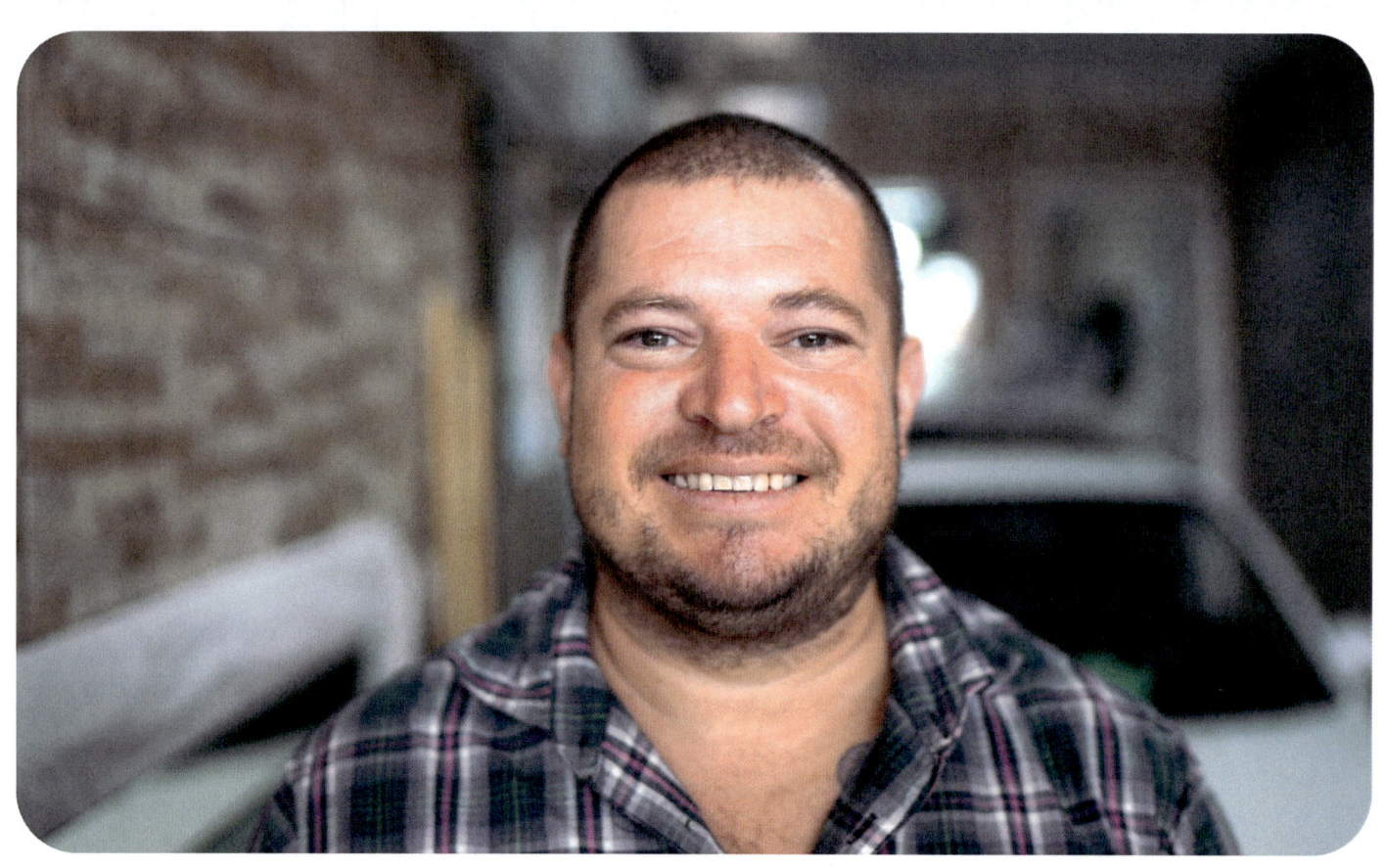

3 Family health history | History with high risk

Colorectal cancer doesn't run in most families. About 1 in 3 people with colorectal cancer have a family member who's had it too. The family history raises your risk, but it doesn't mean that you are certain to get colorectal cancer.

History with high risk

In some families, multiple blood relatives have colorectal cancer. When the cancer occurs in younger or multiple distant relatives, it may be due to a hereditary cancer syndrome.

Hereditary cancer syndromes are caused by an abnormal gene that is passed down from a birth parent to a child. They are rare.

Your health care provider may suspect that you have a hereditary cancer syndrome. If so, they will refer you to an expert in genetics. These experts diagnose and plan management of hereditary cancer syndromes.

There are several types of hereditary cancer syndromes that put a person at high risk of colorectal cancer:

- Lynch syndrome is caused by an inherited error (mutation) in mismatch repair (MMR) genes. Sometimes, Lynch syndrome is referred to as hereditary non-polyposis colorectal cancer (HNPCC), but they are not exactly the same.
- Polyposis syndromes are a group of cancer syndromes that cause multiple colorectal polyps. The most common is familial adenomatous polyposis (FAP).

Know your family history

A family history is one of the most important risk factors for colorectal cancer. Be prepared to tell your health care provider the following information:

- The type of cancer, if any, among blood relatives
- Their age at cancer diagnosis
- Their current age or age at time of death
- Inherited health conditions and birth defects in your family

"

My genetic testing, which identified me with an MSH2 mutation (Lynch syndrome), helped me make decisions about future treatment and understand my future risk for other cancers. This allowed me an opportunity to be proactive in my own healthcare.

– Wenora, Three-time cancer survivor

NCCN Guidelines for Patients®
Colorectal Cancer Screening, 2021

3 Family health history | History with increased risk

Blood relatives

Blood relatives are family members who are related to you by birth. The health history of your blood relatives is important for deciding your risk for colorectal cancer. You share about half (50%) of your genes with first-degree relatives. One-quarter (25%) of your genes are shared with second-degree relatives. You and third-degree relatives share 12.5% of genes.

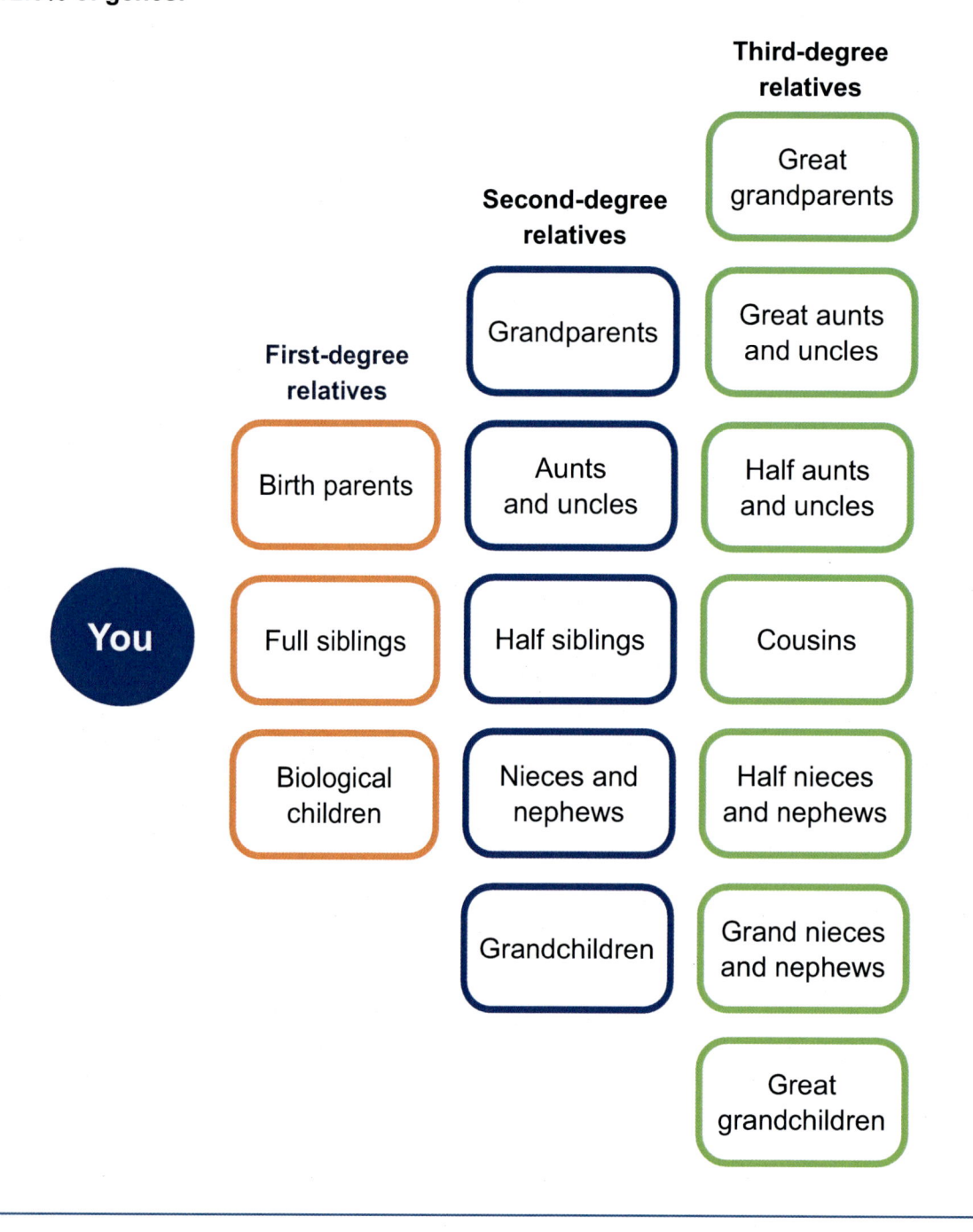

You

First-degree relatives
- Birth parents
- Full siblings
- Biological children

Second-degree relatives
- Grandparents
- Aunts and uncles
- Half siblings
- Nieces and nephews
- Grandchildren

Third-degree relatives
- Great grandparents
- Great aunts and uncles
- Half aunts and uncles
- Cousins
- Half nieces and nephews
- Grand nieces and nephews
- Great grandchildren

NCCN Guidelines for Patients®
Colorectal Cancer Screening, 2021

3 Family health history | History with increased risk

History with increased risk

Most families with a history of colorectal cancer do not have a hereditary cancer syndrome. In these families, the cause of cancer is not clear. The cancer may be caused by shared genes, shared experiences, or both.

Family history of colorectal cancer
You are at increased risk of colorectal cancer if a blood relative has had colorectal cancer. A genetic cause is likely if many relatives have had colorectal cancer. It is also more likely if their cancer occurred before 45 years of age.

Family history of adenoma
Your risk is increased if a first-degree relative has had an advanced adenoma. An adenoma is a common type of polyp.

An advanced adenoma has one or more of these three features:

- High-grade dysplasia – Dysplasia is a pattern of abnormal cell growth. High-grade dysplasia consists of cells that are likely to become cancer.

- Large size – An adenoma is large if it is 1 centimeter in size or larger.

- Villous or tubulovillous histology – Tubular adenomas are the most common, but villous and tubulovillous adenomas are more likely to become cancer. Traditional serrated adenomas (TSAs) have a villous growth pattern.

Family history of sessile serrated polyp
Your risk is increased if a first-degree relative has had a sessile serrated polyp (SSP). An SSP is one of several types of polyps that

---

Growth patterns of adenomas

Adenomas have 3 growth patterns. In tubular adenomas, the glands have a rounded shape (left). Villous adenomas have long glands (middle). Tubulovillous adenomas are a mix of both glands (right).

Tubular: https://commons.wikimedia.org/wiki/File:Tubular_adenoma_2_intermed_mag.jpg
Villous adenoma: https://commons.wikimedia.org/wiki/File:Villous_adenoma1.jpg
Tubulovillous adenoma: https://commons.wikimedia.org/wiki/File:Tubulovillous_adenoma.jpg

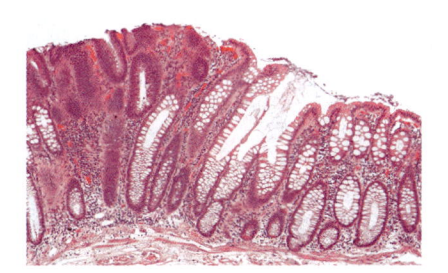

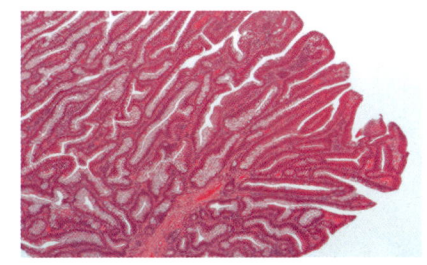

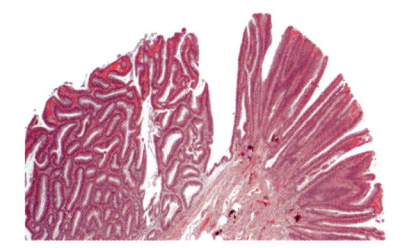

3 Family health history | Key points

have a saw-tooth (serrated) cell pattern. Like adenomas, SSPs have an increased risk of cancer. An advanced SSP has one or both of these two features:

> Dysplasia – An SSP can have a pocket (foci) of dysplasia. These polyps are called sessile serrated polyps with dysplasia (SSP-d).

> Large size – An SSP is large if it is 1 centimeter in size or larger.

Increased-risk screening
Compared to average-risk screening, screening based on family history often starts earlier and is more frequent. **See Guide 3** for screening based on family history.

Your screening schedule can be tailored to you. If there were no concerns on 2 or more prior screenings, the time between screenings may be lengthened. Other factors that may alter screening include your age and the number and age of affected family members.

If you get pre-cancer polyps or colorectal cancer, read Chapter 4 to learn about the next steps.

You can help your family by telling them your screening results. Your doctor may be able to provide test results or a letter that you can share. When your family knows your history, they can make informed decisions for themselves.

Key points

> Lynch syndrome and polyposis syndromes are very rare health conditions that run in families. They are high-risk conditions for colorectal cancer.

> Colorectal cancer screening most often starts before age 40 if your family has colorectal cancer or pre-cancerous polyps but no hereditary cancer syndrome. You may be rescreened in as soon as 5 years even if no polyps are found.

> Since family history affects timing of cancer screening, tell your family about your screening results. They will then be able to make informed decisions for themselves.

Show you care and share your screening results with your family.

NCCN Guidelines for Patients®
Colorectal Cancer Screening, 2021

| 3 | Family health history | Key points |

Guide 3. Screening based on family history

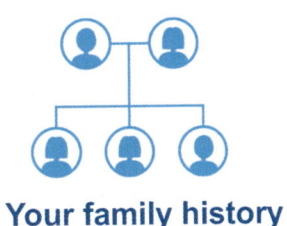

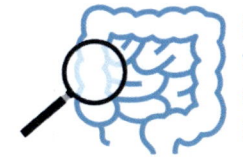

Your family history	Start screening with a colonoscopy at the earlier of the two time points		Time until rescreen if prior results are normal
One or more of your first-degree relatives have had colorectal cancer	Age 40 or	10 years before the first diagnosis of your relatives	Rescreen every 5 years
One or more of your second- and third-degree relatives have had colorectal cancer	Age 45 or	Before age 45 if a relative's cancer had an early onset	Rescreen every 10 years
One or more of you first-degree relatives have had an advanced adenoma or advanced sessile serrated polyp	Age 40 or	Same age as your relative's age at diagnosis	Rescreen every 5 to 10 years

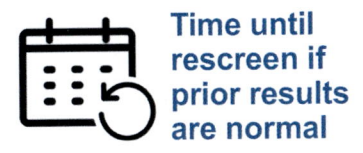

Serrated polyps

Serrated polyps have a saw-tooth cell pattern. There are 3 main types of serrated polyps. Hyperplastic polyps are serrated, and most don't pose a risk of cancer. Sessile serrated polyps may become cancer (shown). Traditional serrated adenomas are rare and may become cancer.

Serrated: https://commons.wikimedia.org/wiki/File:Sessile_serrated_adenoma_2_intermed_mag.jpg

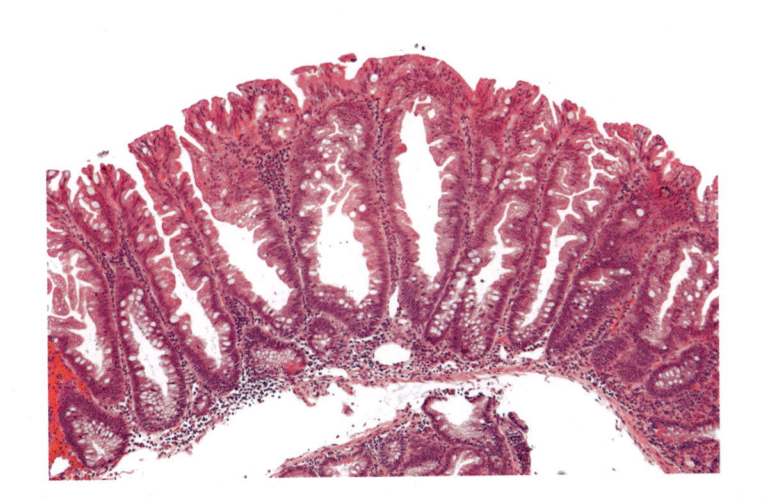

4
Colorectal polyps and cancer

27 Polyps that increase risk
29 Time until rescreening
31 Colorectal cancer
32 Key points

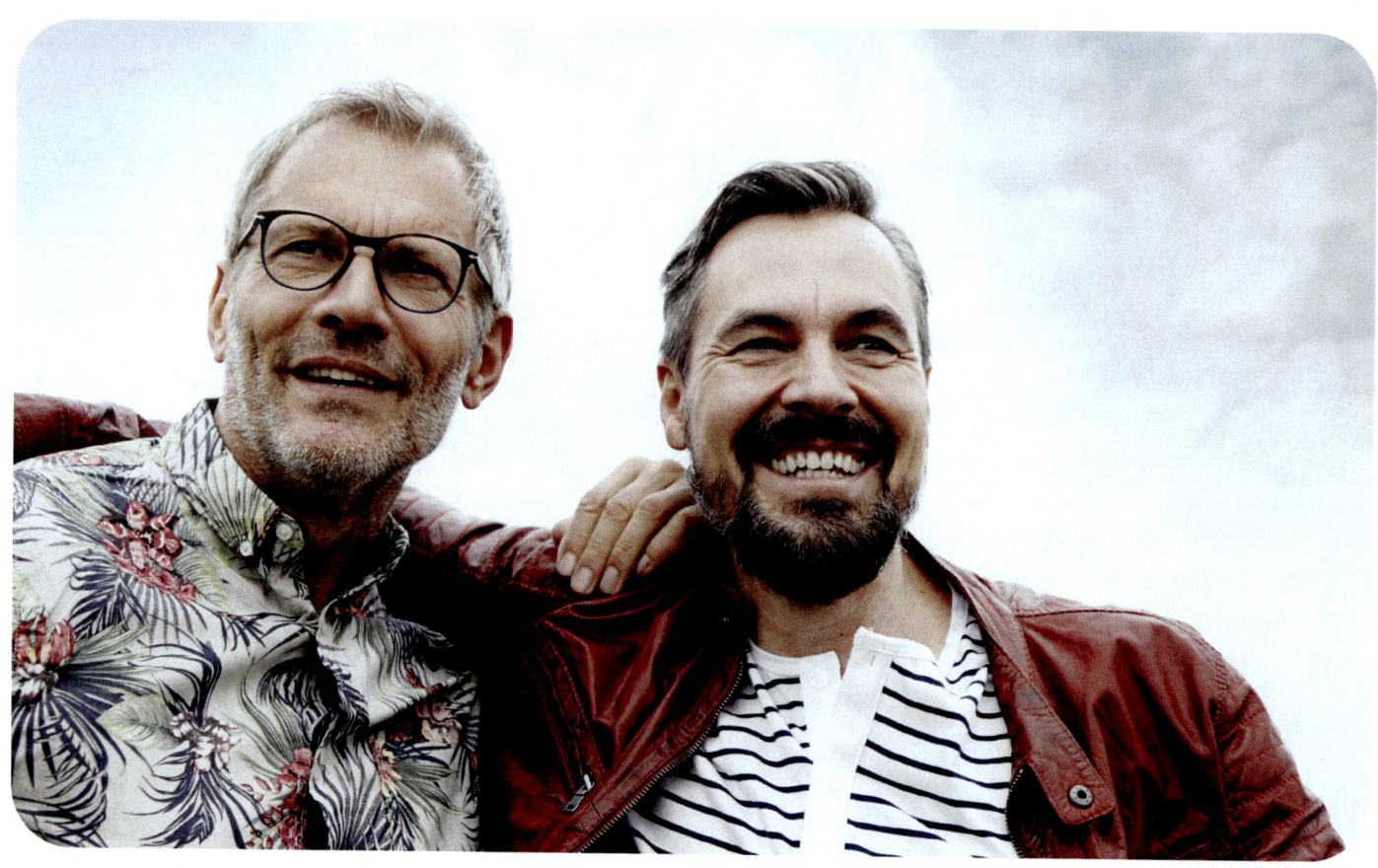

4 Colorectal polyps and cancer | Polyps that increase risk

A colorectal polyp is an overgrowth of the inner lining of the large intestine. Removed polyps are sent to a pathologist to study. The next steps of care are based on what your doctor saw during the colonoscopy and the pathologic findings.

Polyps that increase risk

Most polyps do not become cancer, but your cancer risk is increased if you've had one or more of these three polyps:

Adenoma

An adenoma is also called an adenomatous polyp, traditional polyp, and conventional polyp. It is the most common type of colorectal polyp. It is an overgrowth of gland-like cells that make mucus.

Some adenomas are more likely to become cancer than others. These are called "advanced" adenomas. An advanced adenoma has one or more of these three features:

- High-grade dysplasia – High-grade dysplasia consists of cells that are likely to become cancer.
- Large size – An adenoma is large if it is 1 centimeter in size or larger.
- Villous or tubulovillous histology – Adenomas have 3 types of growth patterns called tubular, villous, and tubulovillous. The tubular pattern is the most common, but villous and tubulovillous adenomas are more likely to become cancer.

Sessile serrated polyp

A sessile serrated polyp (SSP) is raised above the colorectal wall and has a saw-tooth cell pattern. Advanced SSPs have an increased risk of becoming cancer. An advanced SSP has one or both of these two features:

- Dysplasia – An SSP can have a pocket (foci) of dysplasia. These polyps are called sessile serrated polyps with dysplasia (SSP-d).
- Large size – An SSP is large if it is 1 centimeter in size or larger.

Traditional serrated adenoma

Traditional serrated adenomas (TSAs) are rare. They have a villous growth pattern and a saw-tooth cell pattern. They can develop dysplasia. If you've had a TSA, you are likely to get another polyp that has a high risk of becoming cancer.

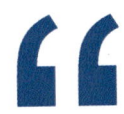

"

We are all very busy with our personal and professional lives. However, colorectal cancer screening is quick and easy and, if completed in a timely manner, can mean the difference between life and death.

– Evan, Rectal cancer survivor

4 Colorectal polyps and cancer | Polyps that increase risk

Polyps found by colonoscopy

Certain features of pre-cancer polyps suggest an increased risk of colorectal cancer. Some features, such as polyp size and shape, can be seen during a colonoscopy. Other features are seen with a microscope.

Shape
Polyps that don't have a stalk are harder to remove and are more likely to become cancer.

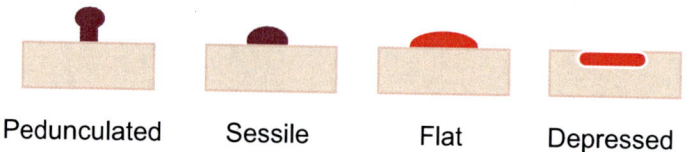

Pedunculated   Sessile   Flat   Depressed

Type
Not all polyps have a risk of cancer. Polyps that may become cancer include adenomas (left) and serrated polyps (right).

Photo credits: Villous adenoma: commons.wikimedia.org/wiki/File:Villous_adenoma1.jpg (left). Serrated polyp: commons.wikimedia.org/wiki/File:Sessile_serrated_adenoma_2_intermed_mag.jpg (right).

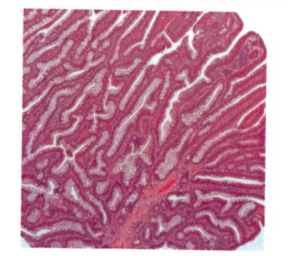

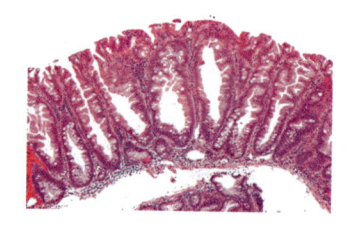

Size
There is a high risk of cancer if polyps are 1 centimeter or larger in size.

½ centimeter Pea   1 centimeter Blueberry   2 centimeters Grape

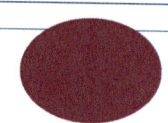

Number
There is a high risk of cancer if there are 3 or more polyps.

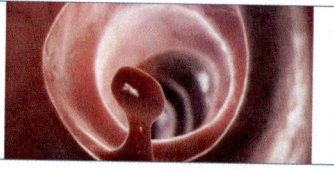

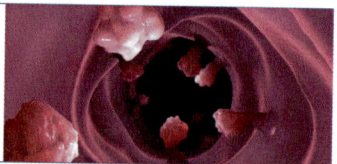

Location
Polyps in the ascending colon have a greater risk of cancer (left). Small hyperplastic polyps in the proximal colon may need more screening (right).

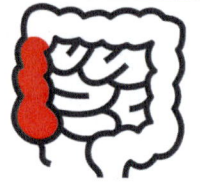

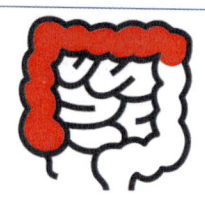

Ascending   Proximal

Dysplasia
Dysplasia is a pattern of abnormal growth. High-grade dysplasia is more abnormal looking than low-grade dysplasia.

Photo credits: Normal colon: commons.wikimedia.org/wiki/File:Colon,_intermed._mag.jpg (left). Low-grade dysplasia: commons.wikimedia.org/wiki/File:Tubular_adenoma_-_colon,_intermed._mag.jpg (middle). High-grade dysplasia: commons.wikimedia.org/wiki/File:Colon_adenoma_with_high-grade_dysplasia,_intermed._mag.jpg (right).

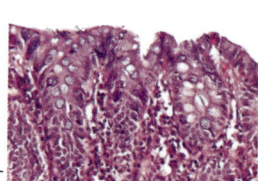

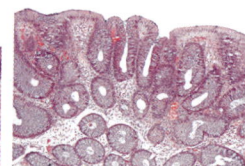

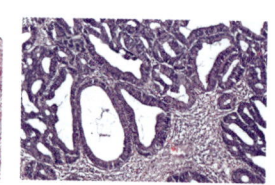

Normal colon   Low-grade dysplasia   High-grade dysplasia

4 Colorectal polyps and cancer | Time until rescreening

Guide 4. Rescreening after removal of small pre-cancer polyps

Number and type of polyp that was removed	Time until rescreening with colonoscopy	If rescreening results are normal, the time until the next screen is extended
1 or 2 adenomas	7 to 10 years	10 years
1 or 2 sessile serrated polyps	5 years	10 years
Traditional serrated adenoma	3 years	5 years
1 or 2 advanced adenomas (high-grade dysplasia, villous or tubulovillous histology)	3 years	5 years
1 to 2 sessile serrated polyps with dysplasia	3 years	5 years
3 to 10 adenomas or sessile serrated polyps	3 years	5 years
11 or more adenomas or sessile serrated polyps	1 to 3 years	The high number of polyps suggests that you have a polyposis syndrome. If genetic testing shows you do not or isn't done, get rescreened.

Time until rescreening

When one or two small adenomas are found and removed, time until rescreening is similar to average risk. If another polyp were to grow, it would take many years for it to become cancer. The risk of a polyp recurrence is greater for serrated polyps, so the interval is shorter. **See Guide 4** for screening intervals after small polyps have been found and removed.

A high number of polyps is a concern. Having 3 to 10 polyps increases your risk of cancer even if the polyps are not advanced. Having more than 11 polyps may be due to a hereditary cancer syndrome. Your doctor should refer you for genetic testing.

NCCN Guidelines for Patients®
Colorectal Cancer Screening, 2021

4 Colorectal polyps and cancer | Time until rescreening

Guide 5. Rescreening after removal of large pre-cancer polyps

Type of polyp that was removed	Time until rescreening with colonoscopy	If rescreening results are normal, the time until the next screen is extended
Pedunculated polyp	3 years	
A sessile, flat, or depressed polyp without additional features for concern	1 to 3 years	3 years
A sessile, flat, or depressed polyp: • Has an increased risk of recurrence • Was removed in pieces	6 months / 1 year	3 years
A sessile, flat, or depressed polyp: • Has risk factors of invasive cancer • Was not fully removed	You may be referred to an endoscopic expert of large polyps or referred to a surgeon	

Large polyps can be hard to remove and may have other features that increase risk of colorectal cancer. In these cases, screening will occur more often or you will be referred to doctors who are experts in removing large polyps. **See Guide 5** for screening intervals after large polyps have been found and removed.

Typically, hyperplastic polyps do not progress into cancer. Doctors are studying whether large hyperplastic polyps do progress into cancer. Hyperplastic polyps are serrated and may be treated like sessile serrated polyps if they are large.

If there is a recurrence, your gastroenterologist may remove the polyp or refer you to another doctor who specializes in colorectal polyps.

4 Colorectal polyps and cancer | Colorectal cancer

Colorectal cancer

About 1 in 24 people in the United States will get colorectal cancer. If you have had colorectal cancer, you have an increased risk for a new (second) colorectal cancer. This risk is not referring to a return of the first cancer, which is called a recurrence. This risk is for a new polyp that will become cancer over time.

For information on cancer surveillance, see *NCCN Guidelines for Patients: Colon Cancer* or *Rectal Cancer* at NCCN.org/patientguidelines. These guidelines also discuss biomarker testing of microsatellite instability (MSI) for all people who have had colorectal cancer. If the cancer cells have MSI, you should also be tested for Lynch syndrome. Having Lynch syndrome increases the risk of colorectal cancer.

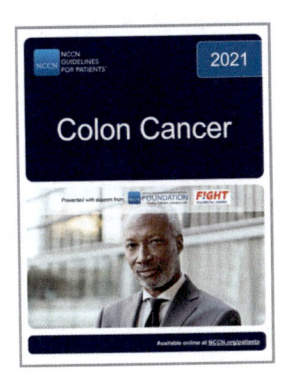

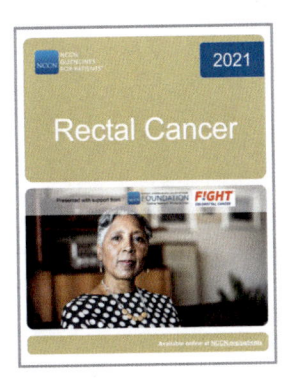

Scientists have learned a great deal about cancer. As a result, today's treatments work better than treatments in the past. Also, many people with cancer have more than one treatment choice.

Who is most affected?

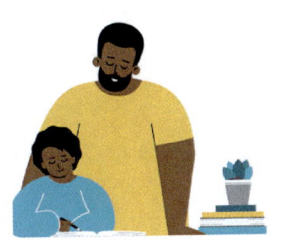

In the United States, Black individuals are more likely to get colorectal cancer, be diagnosed at a young age, and die from the cancer than any other racial or ethnic group.

In addition, Black individuals face many barriers to colorectal cancer screening.

You can take steps to get screened and reduce your risk of colorectal cancer:

- ✓ Start the conversation early. Before age 45, discuss your risk of colorectal cancer with your health care provider.
- ✓ Know your family history of colorectal cancer, which may require earlier screening.
- ✓ Learn about the many acceptable options for colorectal cancer screening.
- ✓ Start screening on time and stay on schedule for follow-up screening.
- ✓ Eat foods that protect against colorectal cancer and avoid unhealthy foods.

4 Colorectal polyps and cancer | Key points

Key points

- You are at increased risk of colorectal cancer if you have had certain polyps. These include adenomas and sessile serrated polyps.

- After these polyps are removed, the timing of the next screening will be based on several factors, such as number of polyps. The timing will also based on if the polyps have abnormal-looking cells, are not fully removed, or have high-risk features.

- If you have had colorectal cancer, you have an increased risk of getting a new cancerous polyp. Follow surveillance recommendations in treatment guidelines.

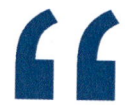

> " A colonoscopy allowed my doctors to solve my mystery ailment. Hearing the words "you have cancer" is life changing. But having my stage II colorectal cancer caught early saved my life.
>
> – Heather

5 Inflammatory bowel disease

34 Chronic inflammation and cancer
35 Start of cancer screening
35 Time until rescreening
37 Key points

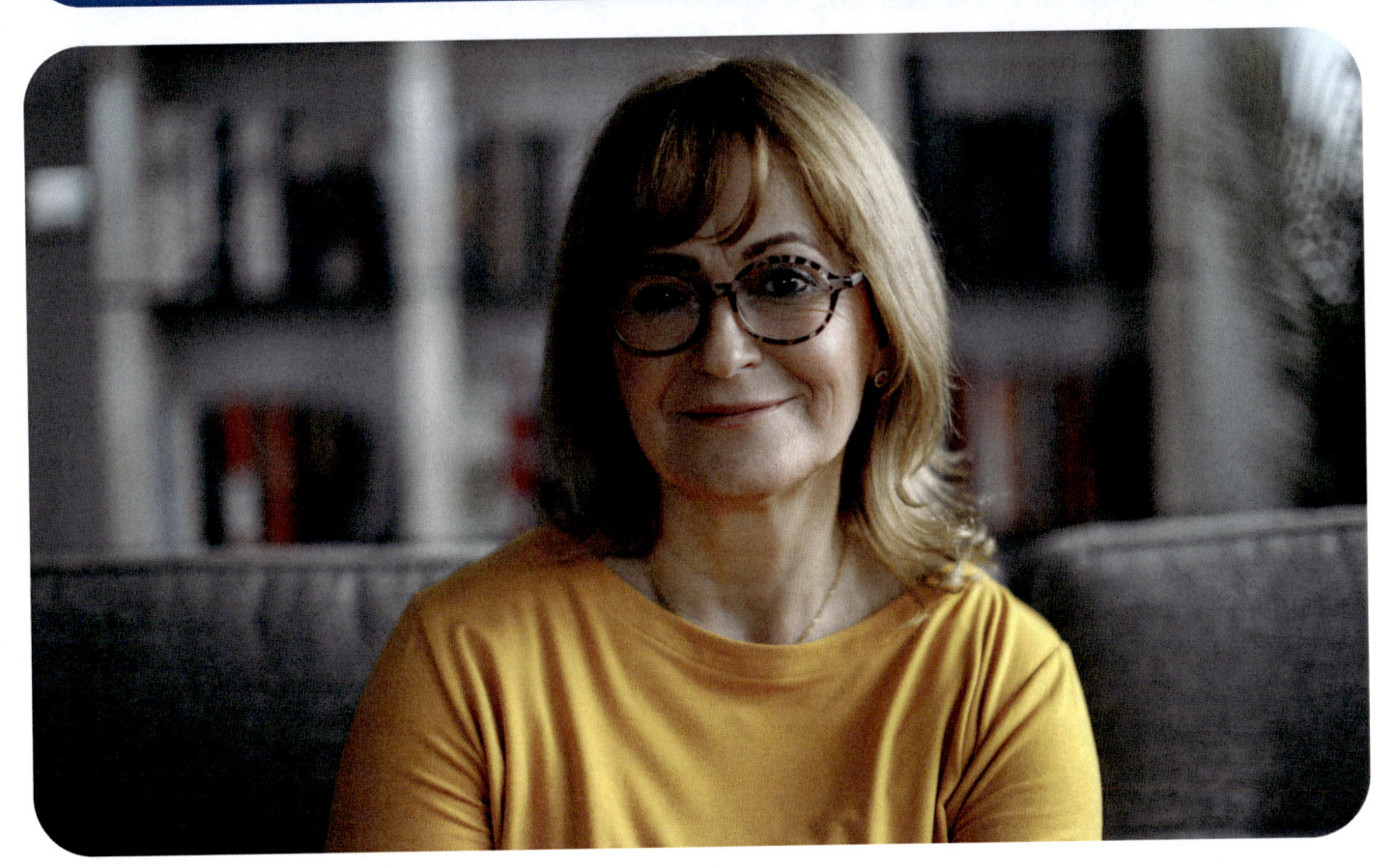

5 Inflammatory bowel disease | Chronic inflammation and cancer

Inflammatory bowel disease causes long-term inflammation and damage within the digestive tract. Two types of this disease that often lead to colorectal cancer are Crohn's colitis and ulcerative colitis.

Chronic inflammation and cancer

Inflammation is a defensive reaction of the body. It occurs when a physical factor triggers the body's immune system. This system sends immune cells to attack the physical trigger. The attack can cause symptoms, such as swelling and pain.

Normal inflammation helps heal the body. Chronic inflammation can cause damage. Chronic inflammation can lead to abnormal cell growth called dysplasia. Dysplasia can become cancer over time.

Inflammatory bowel disease (IBD) is an abnormal response of the immune system to certain cells in the intestinal wall. Crohn's colitis is a type of Crohn's disease that affects the colon. Ulcerative colitis occurs only in the colon and rectum.

Having Crohn's colitis or ulcerative colitis increases your risk of colorectal cancer. Your risk is further increased if you have the following high-risk factors:

- Active or severe, long-lasting inflammation of the colon.

- Inflammation of a large amount of the colon.

- Dysplasia in the colon wall. High-grade dysplasia consists of cells that are likely to become cancer.

- A health condition called primary sclerosing cholangitis, which causes inflammation and narrowing of the bile ducts.

- Blood relatives who have had colorectal cancer, especially if the cancer occurred before 50 years of age.

If you have inflammation that is only in the rectum, you can follow screening for average risk. Read Chapter 2 for screening information.

"

It is important to know colorectal cancer symptoms and know your body. Do not wait or think cancer cannot happen to you.

— Lara, Rectal cancer survivor

NCCN Guidelines for Patients®
Colorectal Cancer Screening, 2021

5 Inflammatory bowel disease | Start of cancer screening

Start of cancer screening

Crohn's disease and ulcerative colitis often start before 30 years of age. There is a second peak of both diseases later in life.

Start colorectal cancer screening at the earliest time point that applies to you:

- 8 years after symptoms of IBD start
- Earlier than 8 years if your family history includes colorectal cancer
- This year if you have primary sclerosing cholangitis

Dysplasia is hard to see because it often occurs in a flat and normal-looking section of the colon wall. It is ideal to do screening when IBD is inactive using the best methods for seeing the colorectal wall.

The screening procedure should always be a colonoscopy. Your doctor will gently guide a thin device through your anus and into your colon while you are sedated. The three options for IBD are:

- High-definition white light endoscopy (HD-WLE) produces over a million colored dots (pixels) on images of your colon. Images are clearer as the number of pixels rises.
- Dye-spraying chromoendoscopy using a high-definition endoscopy applies a stain to the inner colon wall.
- Virtual chromoendoscopy (VCE) using narrow band imaging does not use dyes and instead filters white light. This method is also called optical VCE.

During screening, at least 32 tissue samples will be removed (biopsied) from four parts of your colon. Your doctor will decide which tissue to remove and will space the biopsies 10 centimeters apart. More samples will be removed of any narrowed areas (strictures), masses on the colon wall, or other abnormal areas.

Additionally, during chromoendoscopy, your doctor will perform targeted biopsies of abnormal-looking tissue that can be seen due to the dye or special lighting.

Time until rescreening

If your last screening detected a stricture, you should be seen by an expert in IBD. Strictures of the colon may have underlying cancer. The next step of care may be colectomy. Colectomy is a surgery that removes all or part of your colon. If surgery is not done, you will need to be rescreened in 1 year.

If no polyps or dysplasia were found, get rescreened in 1 year if you have a high risk of cancer. High-risk features include active inflammation, family history, and primary sclerosing cholangitis. Rescreen in 2 to 3 years if there is a low risk of cancer.

Polyps are often removed during cancer screening. Some polyps may require removal by endoscopic mucosal resection (EMR) or endoscopic submucosal dissection (ESD). During EMR, the polyp is lifted up from the colon wall and removed by a wire loop called a snare. ESD uses a knife-like tool to remove polyps.

5 Inflammatory bowel disease | Time until rescreening

If a polyp wasn't fully removed, you may be referred to a center that specializes in IBD. At the center, the polyp may be removed endoscopically. Otherwise, you may see a surgeon to discuss having a colectomy.

You will be rescreened for colorectal cancer if all polyps were fully removed. Polyps that were removed in pieces or had high-grade dysplasia confer a very high risk of cancer. In these cases, get rescreened in 3 to 6 months. If you have high-risk factors for colorectal cancer, get rescreened in 1 year. You can wait 2 to 3 years if you have no high-risk factors.

Invisible dysplasia can't be seen with an endoscope. It might be found in the random samples removed during white light endoscopy. A pathologist who's an expert in the digestive system can aid diagnosis. If dysplasia is confirmed, you should be seen by an expert in IBD. Next steps of care may be a chromoendoscopy if not done before, surgery, or more frequent screening.

See Guide 6 for rescreening intervals based on IBD.

Guide 6. Rescreening based on inflammatory bowel disease (IBD)

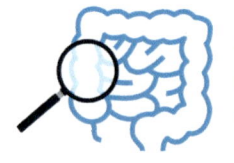

Screening results of prior colonoscopy	Time until rescreening
No polyps or dysplasia were found	• Rescreen in 1 year if you have a minor stricture that wasn't treated with surgery • Rescreen in 1 year if you have high-risk factors • Rescreen in 2 to 3 years if you don't have high-risk factors
"Invisible" dysplasia—can't be seen with an endoscope—was found	• You should be seen by an expert in IBD • You may be rescreened now with chromoendoscopy if not done before • You may be referred to a surgeon
One or more polyps were found	• Rescreen in 3 to 6 months if a polyp was removed in pieces • Rescreen in 3 to 6 months if a polyp had high-grade dysplasia • Rescreen in 1 year if you have high-risk factors • Rescreen in 2 to 3 years if you don't have high-risk factors

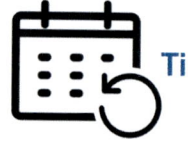

5 Inflammatory bowel disease | Key points

Key points

- People with Crohn's colitis and ulcerative colitis have an increased risk of colorectal cancer.

- The standard time to start colorectal cancer screening is 8 years after IBD symptoms begin. Screening starts earlier if you have a family history or primary sclerosing cholangitis.

- Dysplasia may be hard to see with a typical colonoscopy, so newer methods to see better are used.

- See an IBD expert if you have a stricture or invisible dysplasia, or if an entire polyp wasn't removed. The time until the next screening ranges from 3 months to 3 years based on risk of cancer.

Resources

Colorectal cancer

Fight Colorectal Cancer
FightColorectalCancer.org

National Cancer Institute (NCI)
cancer.gov/types/colorectal

National Comprehensive Cancer Network (NCCN)
Colon Cancer
nccn.org/patients/guidelines/content/PDF/colon-patient.pdf

Rectal Cancer
nccn.org/patients/guidelines/content/PDF/rectal-patient.pdf

Colorectal cancer screening

Fight Colorectal Cancer
fightcolorectalcancer.org/resources/colorectal-cancer-screening

MyPathologyReport
mypathologyreport.ca

National Cancer Institute (NCI)
cancer.gov/types/colorectal/patient/colorectal-screening-pdq

Hereditary cancer syndrome

MedlinePlus
Familial adenomatous polyposis
medlineplus.gov/genetics/condition/familial-adenomatous-polyposis

Lynch syndrome
medlineplus.gov/genetics/condition/lynch-syndrome

Inflammatory bowel disease

Cleveland Clinic
my.clevelandclinic.org/health/diseases/15587-inflammatory-bowel-disease-overview

Survivorship

National Comprehensive Cancer Network (NCCN)
Survivorship Care for Healthy Living
nccn.org/patients/guidelines/content/PDF/survivorship-hl-patient.pdf

Survivorship Care for Cancer-Related Late and Long-Term Effects
nccn.org/patients/guidelines/content/PDF/survivorship-crl-patient.pdf

Words to know

adenoma
An overgrowth of gland-like cells that make mucus. Also called an adenomatous polyp, traditional polyp, and conventional polyp.

anus
An opening through which stool passes out of the body.

biopsy
A procedure to remove tissue or fluid samples to be tested for disease.

blood relatives
People who are related to you by birth.

body mass index (BMI)
A measure of body fat based on height and weight.

colectomy
Surgery to remove a part of the colon.

colon
The hollow organ in which eaten food turns from a liquid into a solid form.

colonoscope
A device that is guided through the anus to work inside the colon.

colonoscopy
A procedure to look inside the colon with a device that is guided through the anus.

computed tomography (CT) colonography
X-rays of the colon.

Crohn's colitis
A health condition that causes long-term swelling in the colon.

Crohn's disease
A health condition that causes long-term swelling in the digestive tract.

depressed polyp
An abnormal growth that lies below the surrounding tissue.

digestive system
A set of organs that changes food into small parts for the body to use as energy.

dye-spraying chromoendoscopy
A procedure to look inside the colon using stains and a device that creates very clear images.

dysplasia
A pattern of abnormal cell growth.

endoscope
A device that is passed through a natural opening to do work inside the body.

endoscopic mucosal resection (EMR)
A procedure that removes growths by lifting then cutting them off with a wire loop that is passed through a natural opening.

endoscopic submucosal dissection (ESD)
A procedure that removes growths with a special knife that is passed through a natural opening.

esophagus
The tube-shaped organ between the throat and stomach.

FAP
familial adenomatous polyposis

fecal immunochemical test (FIT)
A lab test that looks for tiny amounts of blood in stool.

flat polyp
An abnormal growth that does not protrude or slightly protrudes above surrounding tissue.

Words to know

flexible sigmoidoscopy
A procedure to look inside the last part of the colon with a device that is guided through the anus.

high-definition white light endoscopy (HD-WLE)
A procedure to look inside the colon with a device that creates very clear images and is guided through the anus.

high-sensitivity fecal occult blood test
A lab test that looks for tiny amounts of blood in stool.

HNPCC
hereditary non-polyposis colorectal cancer

hyperplastic polyp
An overgrowth of cells that has a saw-tooth cell pattern.

imaging
A test that makes pictures (images) of the inner body.

inflammatory bowel disease
A group of health conditions that cause long-term swelling in the digestive tract.

intestine
The organ that food passes through after leaving the stomach. Also called bowel. It is divided into 2 parts called the small and large intestine.

iron-deficiency anemia
A health condition in which the number of healthy red blood cells is low due to low iron.

laxative
Drugs used to clean out the intestines.

lymph
A clear fluid containing white blood cells.

lymph vessel
A small tube-shaped structure through which a fluid called lymph travels.

Lynch syndrome
A health condition within families that increases the odds of developing cancer.

microsatellite instability (MSI)
Errors made in small, repeated DNA parts during the copy process because of an abnormal repair system.

mismatch repair (MMR) gene
Instructions inside of cells for a protein that corrects DNA errors that occur when DNA copies are being made.

mt-sDNA
multitargeted stool DNA

mucosa
The innermost layer of the colon wall.

multitargeted stool DNA(mt-sDNA)-based test
A lab test that looks for genetic markers of colorectal cancer in stool.

pathologist
A doctor who's an expert in testing cells and tissue to find disease.

pedunculated polyp
An abnormal growth that is shaped like a mushroom.

polyp
An overgrowth of the inner wall of the digestive tract.

polypectomy
A procedure to remove an overgrowth of cells.

polyposis syndromes
A group of health conditions within families that cause multiple colorectal polyps.

Words to know

primary sclerosing cholangitis
A health condition that causes inflammation and narrowing of the bile ducts.

rectum
The hollow organ where stool is held until it leaves the body.

recurrence
A return of a cancer after a cancer-free period.

risk factor
Something that increases the chance of an event.

SD-WLE
standard-definition white light endoscopy

sessile polyp
An overgrowth of cells that has a rounded top and wide base.

sessile serrated polyp (SSP)
An overgrowth of cells with a raised and rounded top and a saw-toothed cell pattern. Also called a sessile serrated adenoma.

sessile serrated polyp with dysplasia (SSP-d)
An overgrowth of cells with a saw-toothed growth pattern and a raised, rounded top.

stool
Unused food that is passed out of the body. Also called feces.

stricture
An abnormal narrowing of a hollow organ.

traditional serrated adenoma (TSA)
An overgrowth of cells that has a saw-tooth cell pattern.

ulcerative colitis
A health condition that causes long-term swelling in the colon or rectum.

virtual chromoendoscopy (VCE)
A procedure to look inside the colon with a light-filtering device that is guided through the anus. Also called optical VCE.

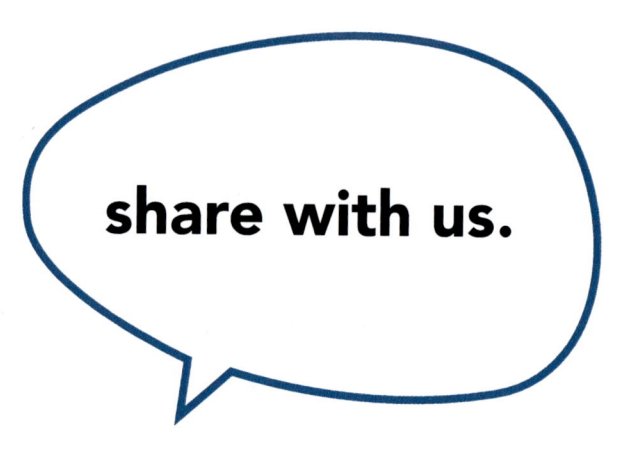

share with us.

Take our survey
And help make the NCCN Guidelines for Patients better for everyone!

NCCN.org/patients/comments

NCCN Contributors

This patient guide is based on the NCCN Clinical Practice Guidelines in Oncology (NCCN Guidelines®) for Colorectal Cancer Screening, Version 2.2021. It was adapted, reviewed, and published with help from the following people:

Dorothy A. Shead, MS
*Senior Director,
Patient Information Operations*

Laura J. Hanisch, PsyD
Patient Information Program Manager

Susan Kidney
Senior Graphic Design Specialist

The NCCN Clinical Practice Guidelines in Oncology (NCCN Guidelines®) for Colorectal Cancer Screening 2.2021 were developed by the following NCCN Panel Members:

Dawn Provenzale, MD, MS/Chair
Duke Cancer Institute

*Reid M. Ness, MD, MPH/Vice Chair
Vanderbilt-Ingram Cancer Center

Benjamin Abbadessa, MD
UC San Diego Moores Cancer Center

Christopher T. Chen, MD
Stanford Cancer Institute

Gregory Cooper, MD
*Case Comprehensive Cancer Center/
University Hospitals Seidman Cancer Center and Cleveland Clinic Taussig Cancer Institute*

Dayna S. Early, MD
Siteman Cancer Center at Barnes-Jewish Hospital and Washington University School of Medicine

*Mark Friedman, MD
Moffitt Cancer Center

Francis M. Giardiello, MD, MBA
The Sidney Kimmel Comprehensive Cancer Center at Johns Hopkins

Kathryn Glaser, MA, PhD
Roswell Park Comprehensive Cancer Center

Suryakanth Gurudu, MD
Mayo Clinic Cancer Center

Amy L. Halverson, MD
Robert H. Lurie Comprehensive Cancer Center of Northwestern University

Rachel Issaka, MD, MAS
*Fred Hutchinson Cancer Center/
Seattle Cancer Care Alliance*

Rishi Jain, MD, MS
Fox Chase Cancer Center

Priyanka Kanth, MD, MS
Huntsman Cancer Institute at the University of Utah

Trilokesh Kidambi, MD
City of Hope National Medical Center

Audrey J. Lazenby, MD
Fred & Pamela Buffett Cancer Center

Xavier Llor, MD, PhD
*Yale Cancer Center/
Smilow Cancer Hospital*

Lillias Maguire, MD
University of Michigan Rogel Cancer Center

Arnold J. Markowitz, MD
Memorial Sloan Kettering Cancer Center

*Folasade P. May, MD, PhD, MPhil
UCLA Jonsson Comprehensive Cancer Center

Robert J. Mayer, MD
Dana-Farber/Brigham and Women's Cancer Center | Massachusetts General Hospital Cancer Center

Shivan Mehta, MD, MBA, MS
Abramson Cancer Center at the University of Pennsylvania

Caitlin Murphy, PhD
UT Southwestern Simmons Comprehensive Cancer Center

Swati Patel, MD, MS
University of Colorado Cancer Center

*Shajan Peter, MD
O'Neal Comprehensive Cancer Center at UAB

*Laura Porter, MD
Patient advocate

Peter P. Stanich, MD
The Ohio State University Comprehensive Cancer Center - James Cancer Hospital and Solove Research Institute

Jonathan Terdiman, MD
UCSF Helen Diller Family Comprehensive Cancer Center

Jennifer M. Weiss, MD, MS
University of Wisconsin Carbone Cancer Center

NCCN Staff

Mallory Campbell, PhD

* Reviewed this patient guide. For disclosures, visit NCCN.org/disclosures.

NCCN Cancer Centers

Abramson Cancer Center
at the University of Pennsylvania
Philadelphia, Pennsylvania
800.789.7366 • pennmedicine.org/cancer

Fred & Pamela Buffett Cancer Center
Omaha, Nebraska
402.559.5600 • unmc.edu/cancercenter

Case Comprehensive Cancer Center/
University Hospitals Seidman Cancer
Center and Cleveland Clinic Taussig
Cancer Institute
Cleveland, Ohio
800.641.2422 • UH Seidman Cancer Center
uhhospitals.org/services/cancer-services
866.223.8100 • CC Taussig Cancer Institute
my.clevelandclinic.org/departments/cancer
216.844.8797 • Case CCC
case.edu/cancer

City of Hope National Medical Center
Los Angeles, California
800.826.4673 • cityofhope.org

Dana-Farber/Brigham and
Women's Cancer Center |
Massachusetts General Hospital
Cancer Center
Boston, Massachusetts
617.732.5500
youhaveus.org
617.726.5130
massgeneral.org/cancer-center

Duke Cancer Institute
Durham, North Carolina
888.275.3853 • dukecancerinstitute.org

Fox Chase Cancer Center
Philadelphia, Pennsylvania
888.369.2427 • foxchase.org

Huntsman Cancer Institute
at the University of Utah
Salt Lake City, Utah
800.824.2073
huntsmancancer.org

Fred Hutchinson Cancer
Research Center/Seattle
Cancer Care Alliance
Seattle, Washington
206.606.7222 • seattlecca.org
206.667.5000 • fredhutch.org

The Sidney Kimmel Comprehensive
Cancer Center at Johns Hopkins
Baltimore, Maryland
410.955.8964
www.hopkinskimmelcancercenter.org

Robert H. Lurie Comprehensive
Cancer Center of Northwestern
University
Chicago, Illinois
866.587.4322 • cancer.northwestern.edu

Mayo Clinic Cancer Center
*Phoenix/Scottsdale, Arizona
Jacksonville, Florida
Rochester, Minnesota*
480.301.8000 • Arizona
904.953.0853 • Florida
507.538.3270 • Minnesota
mayoclinic.org/cancercenter

Memorial Sloan Kettering
Cancer Center
New York, New York
800.525.2225 • mskcc.org

Moffitt Cancer Center
Tampa, Florida
888.663.3488 • moffitt.org

The Ohio State University
Comprehensive Cancer Center -
James Cancer Hospital and
Solove Research Institute
Columbus, Ohio
800.293.5066 • cancer.osu.edu

O'Neal Comprehensive
Cancer Center at UAB
Birmingham, Alabama
800.822.0933 • uab.edu/onealcancercenter

Roswell Park Comprehensive
Cancer Center
Buffalo, New York
877.275.7724 • roswellpark.org

Siteman Cancer Center at Barnes-
Jewish Hospital and Washington
University School of Medicine
St. Louis, Missouri
800.600.3606 • siteman.wustl.edu

St. Jude Children's Research Hospital/
The University of Tennessee
Health Science Center
Memphis, Tennessee
866.278.5833 • stjude.org
901.448.5500 • uthsc.edu

Stanford Cancer Institute
Stanford, California
877.668.7535 • cancer.stanford.edu

UC Davis
Comprehensive Cancer Center
Sacramento, California
916.734.5959 • 800.770.9261
health.ucdavis.edu/cancer

UC San Diego Moores Cancer Center
La Jolla, California
858.822.6100 • cancer.ucsd.edu

UCLA Jonsson
Comprehensive Cancer Center
Los Angeles, California
310.825.5268 • cancer.ucla.edu

UCSF Helen Diller Family
Comprehensive Cancer Center
San Francisco, California
800.689.8273 • cancer.ucsf.edu

University of Colorado Cancer Center
Aurora, Colorado
720.848.0300 • coloradocancercenter.org

University of Michigan
Rogel Cancer Center
Ann Arbor, Michigan
800.865.1125 • rogelcancercenter.org

The University of Texas
MD Anderson Cancer Center
Houston, Texas
844.269.5922 • mdanderson.org

University of Wisconsin
Carbone Cancer Center
Madison, Wisconsin
608.265.1700 • uwhealth.org/cancer

UT Southwestern Simmons
Comprehensive Cancer Center
Dallas, Texas
214.648.3111 • utsouthwestern.edu/simmons

Vanderbilt-Ingram Cancer Center
Nashville, Tennessee
877.936.8422 • vicc.org

Yale Cancer Center/
Smilow Cancer Hospital
New Haven, Connecticut
855.4.SMILOW • yalecancercenter.org

Notes

Index

adenoma 23, 25, 27–29

biopsy 16

chromoendoscopy 35–36

colectomy 35–36

digestive system 7

dysplasia 23–24, 27–29, 34–36

endoscopic mucosal resection (EMR) 35

endoscopic submucosal dissection (ESD) 35

endoscopy 9, 35–36

family history 10–11, 21–25

fecal immunochemical test (FIT) 17–18

flexible sigmoidoscopy 9, 16–19

high-sensitivity fecal occult blood test 18

hereditary cancer syndrome 10, 21, 23, 29

hyperplastic polyp 25, 28, 30

irritable bowel disease (IBD) 10, 34–37

lesion See polyp.

microsatellite instability (MSI) 31

mismatch repair (MMR) gene 21

multitargeted stool DNA (mt-sDNA)–based testing 17–19

polyp 7–8, 10, 27–31, 35–36

polypectomy 16

primary sclerosing cholangitis 34–35

risk 10–11

sessile serrated polyp (SSP) 23, 25, 27–29

symptom 8–9, 12, 21, 34–35

traditional serrated adenoma 23, 25, 27, 29

Made in the USA
Columbia, SC
17 September 2022